Ketogenic Diet

Easy Keto Diet Guide to a Healthy Life and Fast Weight Loss

Heal Yourself and Get More Energy with a Low Carb Diet

Delicious Recipes for Beginners Included

BY SANDRA WILLIAMS

2

Table of Contents

Introduction...5

   [Your Free Gift] 7

Chapter 1: What Is The Ketogenic Diet 10

Chapter 2: Myths Surrounding the Ketogenic Diet 13

Chapter 3: How Does the Ketogenic Diet Work and what are the Benefits of the Diet...15

Chapter 4: What to Eat on the Ketogenic Diet 22

Chapter 5: Side Effects of the Ketogenic Diet................28

Chapter 6: Sample Recipes 30

   Breakfast 30

      Keto Scrambled Eggs 30

      Chocolate Fudge Donuts with Peanut Butter Frosting and Salted Caramel..31

      Steak and Egg Breakfast 34

   Lunch 36

      Keto Pork Chops..36

      Avocado Tuna Melt Bites 38

      Broccoli Chicken Zucchini 40

   Snacks 42

      Cheesy Bacon Bombs 42

Pesto Keto Crackers 44

Savory Pizza Fat Bombs 46

Dinner 47

Caveman Chili 47

Prosciutto, Caramelized Onion, and Parmesan Braid 49

Skilled Browned Chicken with Creamy Greens 53

Dessert 55

Raspberry Fudge Sauce 55

Mexican Chocolate Pudding 56

Salted Almond and Coconut Bark 58

Conclusion 60

Would You Like to Know More? 61

[BONUS] 62

Preview of My Other Book, Wheat Belly Diet 62

Check Out My Other Books 64

Introduction

I want to thank you and congratulate you for purchasing the book *"Ketogenic Diet - Easy Keto Diet Guide For Healthy Life And Fast Weight Loss"*.

Did you know that the United States currently has the highest obesity rates for both children and adults? You could say that this is attributed to our lack of physical activity and our need to eat too much when we do too little. However, I strongly believe that this is a result of our intake of too many carbohydrates. The body only uses what it needs and the rest are stored as fats. I'm not saying that consuming too much protein or fats is good either. However, realistically speaking, it's often harder to consume too much protein or fat because of their filling nature. Carbohydrates, on the other hand are a different ball game, especially refined carbohydrates. Most people eat bread, bagels, doughnuts, cakes, pancakes, waffles, and cookies for breakfast. For lunch, people often choose options like pasta, white rice, and French fries. Potatoes are a common side choice for dinner and maybe some chicken and vegetables. Most often desserts are also full of refined carbohydrates. Can you see what I'm talking about? We are consuming too many carbohydrates! If you want to lose weight, have increased energy levels and restore health, reducing your carbohydrate intake is the solution.

This is what the ketogenic diet is all about. We will look at what exactly the ketogenic diet is, what it entails, how it helps you lose weight, and experience greater energy levels as well as give you some recipes to get started on your journey.

Thanks again for getting this book, I hope you will enjoy it!

PS. This book presents a few recipes, but if you are looking for a full cookbook check out the ***Ketogenic Diet Cookbook*** on Amazon here: http://bit.ly/ketocookbook

[Your Free Gift]

As a way of saying thanks for your purchase, I'm offering 2 free reports that are exclusive to my readers:

To check what are The 101 Tips That Burn Belly Fat Daily go to my page here:

=> http://projecteasylife.com/101tips <=

To see what are The 7 (Quick & Easy) Cooking Tricks To Banish Your Boring Diet go to my website here:

=> http://projecteasylife.com/7-tricks <=

© Copyright 2017 by Sandra Williams - All rights reserved.

This document is geared toward providing exact and reliable information in regards to the topic and issue covered. The publication is sold with the idea that the publisher is not required to render accounting, officially permitted, or otherwise, qualified services. If advice is necessary, legal or professional, consult your health practitioner.

From a Declaration of Principles which was accepted and approved equally by a Committee of the American Bar Association and a Committee of Publishers and Associations.

It's illegal to reproduce, duplicate, or transmit any part of this document either electronically or in print. Recording of this publication is strictly prohibited and any storage of this document is not allowed without written permission from the publisher. All rights reserved.

The information provided herein is stated to be truthful and consistent, in that any liability, in terms of inattention or otherwise, by any usage or abuse of any policies, processes, or directions contained within is the solitary and utter responsibility of the recipient reader. Under no circumstances will any legal responsibility or blame be held against the publisher for any reparation, damages, or monetary loss due to the information herein, either directly or indirectly.

Respective authors own all copyrights not held by the publisher.

The information herein is offered for informational purposes solely, and is universal as so. The presentation of the information is without contract or any type of guarantee assurance.

The trademarks that are used are without any consent, and the publication of the trademark is without permission or backing by the trademark owner. All trademarks and brands within this book are for clarifying purposes only and are owned by the owners themselves, not affiliated with this document.

DISCLAIMER: The purpose of this book is to provide information only. The information, though believed to be entirely accurate, is NOT a substitution for medical, psychological or professional advice, diagnosis or treatment. The author recommends that you seek the advice of your physician or other qualified health care provider to present them with questions you may have regarding any medical condition. Advice from your trusted, professional medical advisor should always supersede information presented in this book.

Chapter 1: What Is The Ketogenic Diet

If you're reading this, chances are you may have come across the word "ketogenic diet" when researching low carb diets. People are increasingly inquiring about this topic: are low carb diets all ketogenic? Is that a good or bad thing? What makes up a ketogenic diet? What are its pros and cons? The biggest factor that determines whether a diet is ketogenic is the amount of carbohydrates. While a moderate reduction of carbohydrates can be very helpful to many people, it won't be ketogenic. To understand the ketogenic diet, it's important to understand ketosis. You may have heard that it's a dangerous state for your body, and it does sound anomalous to be "in ketosis." What it merely means is that your body is using fat for energy.

During fat metabolism, certain molecules known as ketones are generated, whether from the fatty ice cream you just ate, or the fat you are storing around your middle. When your body is breaking down fats for energy, most is converted directly to ATP (adenosine triphosphate). Ketones are produced as by-products of the process. When you eat fewer carbohydrates, your body relies on fat for energy, so it makes sense why more ketones are produced. Some of those ketones are used for energy, namely acetoacetate and ß-hydroxybutyrate. The kidneys and the heart muscles particularly prefer ketones to glucose. Also, many of our body cells, including brain cells, can use ketones for some of their energy. However, one kind of ketone molecule known as acetone cannot be used for energy, and is eliminated as waste, usually through breathing and urine.

If there's enough acetone in your urine, you can use a dipstick commonly referred to as Ketostix to detect it, although there are other brands. While everyone is continuously generating ketones, their detection in the urine is what's usually referred to as ketosis. The more ketones there are in the urine, the darker the stick turns purple. The Atkins diet especially advises people to check their ketosis as a sign of fat burning. Other low carb diets don't pay much attention to this, or aren't low enough in carbohydrates to make much of an impression on the sticks.

So, basically, a ketogenic diet is one that puts your body in ketosis where you burn fat for energy by reducing your carbohydrate intake greatly so that your body uses fat instead. This means that a ketogenic diet can be very effective in helping you burn fat. Despite this, some people still think that ketosis is so bad. Why is this so?

There is a general assumption that if your body is burning plenty of fat for energy, it must not be getting sufficient glucose. However, studies of people on reduced carbohydrate diets show no indication that this is true. Although our bodies cannot break down fat into glucose, we can convert some of the protein we eat into glucose. This is very convenient for those who cannot tolerate a lot of sugar, especially because this conversion takes place slowly, ensuring that it doesn't spike blood sugar levels. Therefore, you need to understand that the ketosis produced because of limiting carbohydrate intake or fasting doesn't have negative effects in most people once they've adapted to that state.

The main concern arises from the fact that people who are unable to produce insulin, mainly those with type 1 and 2 diabetes, can get into a dangerous state known as diabetic ketoacidosis. In this state, the level of ketones is generally higher than that in ketosis. The ketosis brought about by diet has been called dietary ketosis, benign dietary ketosis, physiological ketosis, and nutritional ketosis most recently in a bid to clear up any confusion with ketoacidosis. The second source of confusion involves the transition period where the body takes some time to adapt to using ketones and fats, as opposed to glucose as its main source of energy. During this period, there can be negative symptoms such as fatigue, light-headedness, mild irritability, headaches, and weakness. The good news is that most of these are over within the first week of the diet, although some may go well into the second week.

There have been many misconceptions about the ketogenic diet, so let us look at these myths and set the facts straight.

Chapter 2: Myths Surrounding the Ketogenic Diet

A low carb diet is not good for your kidneys

This myth came about because when you have kidney problems, you're usually advised to reduce your protein intake. Since people believe that a ketogenic diet is high in protein, they assume that it's unhealthy if you have kidney problems. However, this isn't the case. The ketogenic diet is high in fat but not necessarily high in protein.

High intake of fats can cause heart attack

If you eat a diet high in carbohydrates as well as fats, fat will definitely be stored, and carbohydrates will be used for energy. The excess fats can increase the body fat ration and clog the arteries, which may lead to many complications. However, on the ketogenic diet, you reduce your carbohydrate intake and increase fat consumption; hence, the body turns to burning fat for energy, so there's no accumulation.

Glucose is the only fuel that the brain can use

This is very incorrect since brain cells are flexible and can derive energy from glucose as well as ketone bodies. Even though the brain may still require some glucose to function adequately, most of the fuel can come from ketones, which are usually made from fatty acids.

A Ketogenic diet is not suitable for building muscle

This myth is quite laughable considering that many athletes have already adapted to the ketogenic diet. What you need to understand is that you don't have to take huge amounts of carbohydrates to build muscle; actually, you need more protein. While you need glucose to transport the protein into the muscle, you don't need too much glycogen. The carbohydrates from proteins, fats and vegetables are enough.

Now that we have cleared some of the common misconceptions about ketogenic diet, let us look at how the ketogenic diet works.

Chapter 3: How Does the Ketogenic Diet Work and what are the Benefits of the Diet

What would you say if I told you that you could boost your energy levels with only a change in your diet? What about losing fat with the same diet? How would you fancy eating the foods that are generally considered a taboo? The good foods… you know, the ones with all fats that taste amazing. We are talking about the ketogenic diet. Countless books have been written about this very topic, and yet most of the population is ignorant of its value. The same comments still linger "Man, that diet is not good for you," "You will gain too much cholesterol and probably get a heart attack." What is the root of all this? A common lack of knowledge! It's human nature for us to fear what we don't understand, which is why you're here to gain some ground on the subject, and probably end up with a better understanding of the diet.

The objective of the diet is to force your body into a glycogen deprived state, and stay that way while maintaining a mild state of ketosis (converting fat into energy). For this to happen, you need to minimize the carbohydrates in your diet and increase your fat intake. Carbohydrates are converted into glucose on a carb-based diet, and this is what your body normally uses as its primary fuel source. The excess glucose is converted into glycogen and then stored in your liver for future use. Once your stores are full, you experience some sort of spill over, and the extra is stored as fat or adipose tissue, as you are probably familiar with.

If you feel like you don't eat a lot, but still get fat, it is probably because of an insulin intolerance. You'd be shocked by the number of people who are borderline pre-diabetic. How many obese people do you know today? If you asked some of them what makes up their meals, and how much they eat, I guarantee you would be surprised by their answers. Most people are struggling with weight due to insulin intolerance, especially as the aging process takes toll. The most interesting thing about this factor is that you can control this insulin complication by using this diet.

There are several carbohydrate-related problems we are dealing with today, including diabetes, high blood pressure, and heart disease, which are primarily caused by hyper-insulinism. Scientists have discovered in the last 10 to 15 years that metabolic complications that normally occur in the obese are caused by insulin resistance. The insulin hormone is constantly rising and falling, depending on the foods you eat. Thus, managing your carbohydrate intake is also suitable in managing various health conditions.

Optimal ketosis?

So, how do you get to a state of optimal ketosis when your body simply burns fat and insulin levels are at their lowest? The trick is to avoid all possible carbs and keep your protein intake moderate (just to ensure that your body doesn't start breaking proteins to glucose since this likely raises insulin levels). You don't want that to happen if you're trying to get your body to its highest state of burning fat. A great way of ensuring that you achieve this is consuming more fat; it could be taking such things like magic bullet coffee (this usually entails adding a tablespoon of coconut oil and a tablespoon of butter to your morning coffee then blending the mix). This should keep your carb and protein cravings at bay. This will push your body to an optimal ketosis state, especially with zero carb and moderate protein intake. You'll need anywhere between 2-7 days to get into optimal ketosis based on your activity level, body type, and what you eat. A good way to help you reduce the time it takes to get into the state of optimal ketosis is to exercise on an empty stomach, then keep carb intake to 20g or less. This is where the ketogenic diet comes into play!

Let's look at how you can benefit by embracing the ketogenic diet:

Increased energy levels

You may not believe this, but glucose isn't your body's favorite fuel source. We constantly subject it to carbohydrates, and the problem is that carbohydrates aren't efficient or clean burning. Suppose your body was a car. Would you rather fill its tank with the lowest grade gas when it requires the higher grade? What would be the result? Dirty valves, lousy gas mileage, pinging, and soon the remaining power would slow down.

The same applies to your body. After a few days of carbohydrate withdrawal, most people report increased energy levels to the point where they can literally bounce off the walls. With the huge density of nutritional energy in one gram of fat, is it a wonder? Your body's actual preferred fuel source is free form fatty acids. However, with carbohydrate-based diets, your body scarcely gets the chance to use them, mainly because glucose is more readily available and easier to utilize. Your body will assume the easiest method, which may not necessarily be the best energy method. It's very simple. If you consume carbohydrates, it will use carbohydrates. On the contrary, if you feed it fats, it will use fats. The mechanism behind this fact is that it actually takes less energy to burn carbohydrates as opposed to fats, which are 4 calories per gram and 9 calories per gram respectively. Therefore, unless you force your body to utilize fatty stores in the first place, it will not.

Decreased hunger while slimming

It's not complicated, really. Fat has more nutritional density than carbohydrates. Fat takes a longer time to digest, which leaves you feeling fuller for longer. It's like your body is telling you that it's happy and satisfied. On the other hand, when you eat a carbohydrate-based meal, you tend to feel hungry a short time later. The rapid boost in insulin will result to a couple of things. It will lead to increased lethargy, i.e. feeling excessively tired, and will leave you feeling hungry again soon afterward. Have you ever wondered why you feel tired almost immediately after eating a high carb meal, such as a large bowl of pasta? What about one hour later when you find yourself going for a snack again? This is a common scenario with a carb-based diet. It all boils down to the same factor - insulin. To be more specific, it's a chemical disorder known as hyper-insulinism. It occurs largely because of the refined carbohydrates and sugar most people consume today.

Man wasn't meant to consume refined carbohydrates or sugar, and in my opinion, this is what's slowly poisoning us. Can you recall the last time you dieted? Do you remember how you always seem to feel hungry, and how you persevered because you were never satisfied with the meals you ate? You must have had times when you wished you could end your dieting misery and get back to eating. Everyone who has ever tried dieting has passed through this at one time or the other. This is where the keto diet comes into play. Consider this: rich fatty foods to counter your cravings. Sounds tempting, huh?

Unfortunately, not everyone can eat whatever he or she wants and get away with it. A lot of people gain weight while doing so. Why? There could be numerous reasons, but the main reason is eating the wrong foods and ratios. Your body's metabolism rate tends to slow down as you age, and fat becomes a lot easier to gain and keep in your body. You soon discover that a simple food item that you used to eat with little concern now causes you to gain fat. You also realize that your training is affected because you're too tired to workout let alone stand and walk. You eventually find yourself relying on supplements such as ECA (Ephedrine, Caffeine, Aspirin) stacks to carry you through the day. But these stacks only work for a short time, and then you become restless again.

People are constantly struggling to find ways to increase their metabolism to lose excess fat, but they often fail in this quest. In most cases, it's because you're not given a heads up with certain diets. How many have been told that the secret to proper nutrition is to blend your foods and eat carbs, fats, and a small portion of protein at each meal. Have you ever noticed people who lose fat but fail again in the future? The answer is rather simple: they failed to condition their bodies for permanent weight loss. They took on a strict diet for the sole purpose of losing ten pounds in the first week, and then five to six pounds every time thereafter. That's all great, but with calorie deficiency in your diet, and once you reach your goal weight, fat creeps in once again. Thus, blending fats and carbohydrates is a big NO... Why is this?

You're probably aware that carbohydrate intake will boost insulin response, and this is good. When you eat fats and carbohydrates at the same time, the fats will be deposited to the adipose tissue as they try to be drawn up into the body. This is what leads to fatty deposits in your body. This is the problem with obese people. They're not sure how to eat, and eating French fries (fats and carbohydrates), is not the best way to go. Food is a rather powerful drug, and it can either make or break you. It all depends on you. Even bodybuilders tend to make the same mistakes in their diets. It's all too common. You see a trainee trying to cut down by eating a supposed well balanced diet with carbohydrates, fats and proteins, only to have a difficult time losing the fat. You may have heard that you need to eat fats and carbohydrates. Well, the answer is yes, and no.

Yes, if the timing is correct. After all, there is a right and wrong time for everything. When you're young, everything you eat seems to be passing through your system, and no additional weight may be accompanied by eating garbage. That's why you increase your fat intake and decrease carbohydrates on the ketogenic diet for maximum weight loss.

Improved brain health

Carbohydrate restriction triggers the production of fatty acids by the fat cells in the pancreas, which are then taken up by the liver and converted into ketones before being released into the bloodstream. Once the ketones are taken up into your brain, they enter the TCA (the citric acid cycle) to produce energy. So, your brain is happily generating energy from ketones... sure, but how would this help protect you against a variety of brain diseases?

A good answer may be energy. Several neurological diseases, despite their superficial differences, share a common problem i.e. insufficient energy production. Ketones serve as an alternative energy source during metabolic stress to maintain normal brain cell metabolism. Surprisingly, a major ketone known as BHB may even have a higher fuel affinity than glucose, providing you with more energy per unit oxygen used.

The number of mitochondria in the brain also rises while on a ketogenic diet. Hippocampal cells usually degenerate in age related diseases, resulting in cognitive dysfunction and memory loss. Neurons can fight off disease stressors with increased energy reserve, which would otherwise exhaust and kill the cell. A keto diet can also directly hinder a major source of neuronal stress by... well, you know, acting like a blueberry. However, reactive oxygen species are produced as byproducts of cellular metabolism. These oxidants contain a single electron, unlike the gas oxygen, which makes them highly reactive, attacking membranes, proteins, and wrecking their structure. Subsequently increased oxidants are a sign of aging, neuro-degeneration and stroke.

Ketones inhibit the production of these volatile molecules directly and increase the activity of glutathione peroxidase to enhance their breakdown. The low carbohydrate intake also directly minimizes glucose oxidation, something known as glycolysis. One study found that neurons trigger stress proteins to reduce oxidant levels and stabilize the mitochondria. Since the ketogenic diet has high fat content, it increases poly-unsaturated fatty acids such as EPA and DHA, both sold as OTC brain healthy supplements. This then reduces the oxidant production as well as inflammation.

Let us now look at what you can eat while on the ketogenic diet.

Chapter 4: What to Eat on the Ketogenic Diet

Fats and oils

Since dietary fats will be the main energy source, you should make your choices with digestive tolerance in mind. Majority of people cannot tolerate eating a huge amount of olive oil, vegetable oil, or even mayonnaise for a long time. Well, this is actually good, because vegetable oils are packed with polyunsaturated omega 6 fatty acids. You should eliminate omega 6 fatty acids found in canola oil, corn oil, safflower oil, soybean oil, margarines, and nut oils because of their inflammatory effect within the body. Most nuts, except walnuts and macadamias are rich in omega 6 fatty acids too, so don't eat them often.

You should balance your polyunsaturated fat intake between omega 3 and omega 6 types. Eating shellfish, tuna, and salmon provides essential omega 3 fatty acids, which are important to a low carb meal plan. If you don't like seafood, then consider taking small amounts of a krill or fish supplement. Most people can easily tolerate saturated and monounsaturated fats such as egg yolks, avocado, coconut oil, macadamia nuts, and butter. They're also less inflammatory, since they are chemically stable. With time, it will become second nature to add a fat source to every meal.

Steer away from hydrogenated fats like margarine in to minimize trans-fats intake. On the other hand, if you use vegetable oils (sesame, soybean, safflower, sunflower, canola and olive oils), go for the "cold pressed." Preserve the cold pressed oils such as flaxseed and almond in the refrigerator to avoid rancidity. Also, avoid heating vegetable oils, and use clean non-hydrogenated coconut oil, beef tallow, lard, olive oil, and ghee for frying, because these have high smoke points.

Protein

Fattier chunks of meat are better because they have less protein, and obviously more fat. If possible, go for the grass fed or organic animal foods and organic eggs in to minimize antibiotic, bacteria, and steroid hormone intake. Here are the best clean protein choices for a ketogenic diet food list:

Meat: goat, veal, lamb, beef wild game. grass fed meat is the best because it has a better fatty acid profile.

Poultry: quail, turkey, chicken, goose, duck, Cornish hen, and pheasant. Free range is preferred.

Pork: ham, pork chops, Boston butt, and pork loin. Watch out for added sugar in hams.

Fish and seafood: preferably wild caught tuna, trout, snapper, sole, scrod, sardines, salmon, mahi-mahi, mackerel, herring, halibut, flounder, cod, catfish, calamari and anchovies. Canned tuna and salmon are not prohibited, but scan the labels for added fillers or sugars. Shellfish like oysters, mussels, squid, shrimp, scallops, lobster, crab, and clams. Avoid imitation crabmeat, as this contains gluten, sugar, and other additives. Steer clear of breaded and fried seafood.

Whole eggs: You can prepare these in a variety of ways: soft boiled, scrambled, poached, omelets, hard boiled, fried, and deviled.

Bacon and sausage: Read the labels and avoid those treated with sugar or fillers such as wheat or soy. You can find most brands of sugar free bacon in specialty health food stores.

Whey protein powders + hemp, pea, rice, and any other vegetable protein powders.

Fresh vegetables

Majority of the non-starchy vegetables are low in carbohydrates. To avoid pesticide residues, go for organic vegetables or grow your own. Avoid starchy vegetables such as sweet potatoes and potatoes as well as most winter squash because they have more carbohydrates. Minimize your sweet vegetables such as summer squashes, peppers, carrots, and tomatoes.

Some great leafy green vegetables that you can eat include: Bamboo Shoots, Beet Greens, Broccoli, Cabbage, Celery, Chard, Collard Greens, Dandelion Greens, Garlic, Leeks, Mushrooms, Sauerkraut, Shallots, Spinach, Turnips, Alfalfa Sprouts, Asparagus, Bean Sprouts, Brussels Sprouts, Cauliflower, Celery Root, Chives, Cucumbers, Dill Pickles, Kale, Lettuces and salad greens (Bok Choy, Arugula, Boston lettuce, Endive, Chicory, Escarole, Mache, Fennel, Radicchio, Sorrel, Romaine.), Radishes, Scallions, Swiss Chard and Water Chestnuts among many other vegetables.

Dairy products

Raw milk products are better. Some dairy products that are okay include:

- Full fat sour cream (watch out for fillers and additives in the labels.)

- Heavy whipping cream

- Full fat cottage cheese

- Cream cheese

- All hard and soft cheeses

- Mascarpone cheese

- Unsweetened whole yogurt (minimize amounts because it is slightly higher in carbohydrate)

Nuts and seeds

These are best soaked and roasted in to extract the most nutrients. Steer away from peanuts since these are legumes.

Nuts: walnuts, almonds, pecans and macadamias are the lowest in net carbohydrates, and can be consumed in small amounts. Chestnuts, pistachios, and cashews are higher in carbohydrates, so tread carefully to avoid going over carbohydrate limits. Nuts are also richer in omega 6 fatty acids that are inflammatory, so avoid relying on nuts as your main source of protein.

Nut flours, like almond flour. The main reason for including this is that a low carb meal plan should not completely exclude baking. Almond flour is a superb flour substitute.

Beverages

- Decaf coffee

- Herbal tea (unsweetened)

- Flavored seltzer water (unsweetened)

- Clear broth or bouillon

- Decaf tea (unsweetened)

- Water

- Lemon and lime juice in small quantities

Sweeteners

Avoid sweetened foods to reset your taste buds, so to speak. If you have cravings for something sweet, these are the recommended options. Note that most artificial sweeteners in powder form usually contain dextrose, maltodextrin, or some other added sugar, so liquid products are better.

- Stevia, preferably liquid because the powdered usually contains maltodextrin

- Xylitol

- Erythritol

- Monk fruit

- Lo Han Guo

- Splenda, preferably liquid because the powdered form usually contains maltodextrin

- Chicory root and Inulin

Spices

Most people tend to disregard this, but spices do contain carbohydrates, so be sure to count them when adding them to your meals. Commercial spice mixes such as steak seasoning usually contain added sugar. Sea salt is better than commercial salt. Cinnamon, cilantro/coriander seeds, chili pepper, cayenne pepper, black pepper, basil, peppermint, parsley, oregano, mustard seeds, ginger, dill, cumin seeds, cloves, turmeric, thyme, sage and rosemary are some of the amazing spices that are most ideal.

Chapter 5: Side Effects of the Ketogenic Diet

Most people wouldn't refer to the keto diet as a diet. It's more like a nutritional system, learning to live without all the refined sugars, subsequently causing a series of crashes during withdrawal. The ketogenic diet will significantly transform your metabolism as your body starts using all the calories you consume for fuel rather than directing them to fat storages to prevent blood sugar spike. Insulin is what causes weight gain since excess glucose is stored as fat. Without insulin, sugar would kill us. From an evolutionary and biological standpoint, the only time we're supposed to use carbohydrates for calories is as a last resort, to prevent starvation.

Now for the cons:

- The transition period is usually the most difficult part. You have to plan to count your carbohydrates and calories. Consider investing in a carbohydrate free protein powder. This will go a long way toward enabling you to hit your protein and fat percentages (30 percent and 65 percent of calorie intake). Chances are, you will also experience some digestive complications as your body adjusts to the diet. You may also experience lightheadedness and temporary loss of energy during the transition phase. Bad breath is a common beginning side effect due to either insufficient fat and too much protein and/or dehydration.

- Speaking of dehydration, since carbohydrates make your body store water, you probably won't get as much water from carbohydrates. It's usually advisable to drink 8 glasses of water per day, right? However, on the keto diet, you need to drink more water, and this can be challenging, especially if you're not used to drinking 8 glasses of water every day.

- You'll also have to be very keen on your nutrition. With such limited carbohydrate intake and no fruit, it's very easy for your body to deplete on magnesium, potassium, and vitamin C. So, get some carbohydrate free electrolyte powder, take a multivitamin, and be sure to eat a lot of spinach, cauliflower, asparagus, broccoli, and arugula. These are the five staple veggies to count on for nutrition.

- You're also likely to experience massive cravings for sugar and carbohydrates. For most people, this usually happens about a week after starting the diet, and can last up to two weeks. As a result, you may end up with a higher calorie intake.

- In addition, you'll find it much harder to build muscle while on a ketogenic diet. This is primarily because carbohydrates enhance the protein absorption into your muscles, while fat slows it down. The best way to counter this is to eat a few carbohydrates immediately after a workout.

If you can live with those side effects, then the ketogenic diet may be for you. But it's certainly not for everyone. The most difficult challenge is the induction phase after which your life will change in very positive ways. Even within the first few days without carbohydrates, it feels like a curtain of fog has been peeled away, and you suddenly experience real energy.

Chapter 6: Sample Recipes

Breakfast

Keto Scrambled Eggs

(327 calories, 26.52g fat, 1.8g carbs, 18.36g protein)

Serves 1

Ingredients

- 1 T unsalted butter
- 3 large eggs
- Coarse salt and freshly ground pepper

Directions

1. Beat the eggs using a fork. Add the butter to a medium nonstick skillet and melt over low heat. Stir in the egg mixture. Pull the eggs gently to the center of the pan using a heatproof flexible spatula, and leave the liquid parts to run out under the parameter. Continue cooking while moving the eggs with the spatula until set, about 1 ½ to 3 minutes.

2. Add salt and pepper to season, and serve hot with green leafy vegetables of choice.

Chocolate Fudge Donuts with Peanut Butter Frosting and Salted Caramel

(171 calories per serving, 13.3g fat, 5.2g carbs, 2.6g fiber, 2.6g net carbs, 3.6g protein)

Serves 5

Ingredients

- 2 T butter
- 1/4 c granulated erythritol
- 3 T cocoa powder
- 1/2 t instant coffee granules
- 2 T water
- 1 t vanilla extract
- 1/4 t liquid stevia (the kind with the erythritol in it)
- 1 egg
- 2 T coconut flour
- 1/4 t cream of tartar
- 1/4 t baking soda
- 1/4 t xanthan gum

Directions

1. In a small saucepan, combine the butter, erythritol, cocoa and coffee granules. Stir constantly over medium-high until

mixture is smooth and erythritol is completely dissolve. Remove from heat. Stir in water, vanilla extract and stevia. Let cool until just warm, then stir in the egg. Set aside.

2. Sift coconut flour, cream of tartar, baking soda and xanthan gum into a mixing bowl. Pour in wet ingredients and stir until smooth. Transfer to a baggy, cut off the corner. Pipe equally into 5 wells of sprayed donut pan. Bake at 375° for 8 minutes. Turn out onto cooling rack and let cool slightly.

Peanut butter frosting:

- 1 T butter
- 2 T erythritol
- 2 T creamy peanut butter

1. In a small saucepan, combine butter and erythritol. Heat over medium until erythritol is dissolved. Remove from heat, stir in peanut butter. Let cool slightly. Transfer to baggy. Set aside.

Salted caramel drizzle:

- 2 T cold butter, divided
- 1 T dark or light maple syrup
- 1 T erythritol

1. In a small saucepan, combine 1 T butter, erythritol and maple syrup. Over medium-high, stir until bubbly and smooth. Remove from heat. Stir in remaining tablespoon of butter. Let cool. Transfer to baggy, set aside.

2. Cut a corner off the baggy of peanut butter frosting. Pipe onto donuts. Cut the corner off if the baggy of caramel. Drizzle over donuts.

Steak and Egg Breakfast

(606 calories, 46g fat, 4g carbs, 1g fiber, 3g net carbs, 46g protein)

Serves 2

Ingredients

- 8 oz cubed steak
- 4 large egg
- 2 T butter divided
- 2 oz cheddar cheese
- 8 oz trimmed asparagus
- Salt and pepper

Directions

1. Trim the asparagus and place into a microwavable dish. Add 1 tablespoon water and cover with plastic wrap.

2. Cube Steak: Season both sides of cube steak with salt and pepper. Heat a medium sized heat skillet over medium heat. When hot, add one tablespoon of butter and swirl to coat the bottom. Add the seasoned cube steaks and cook 3-41/2 minutes per side (or longer) depending on your cooking preference. (Meanwhile, start cooking the eggs.) Remove the cooked cube steaks and gently cover with foil.

3. Cheesy Scrambled Eggs: While the steaks are cooking, place a medium non-stick pan over medium heat. Crack 4 eggs into a medium bowl and add 2 ounces of grated

cheese. Mix together with a fork. When the pan is hot, add 1 tablespoon of butter and swirl to coat the pan. Add the egg mixture to the pan and leave it alone for a few moments while it cooks on the bottom. Gently scrape the cooked egg to the center of the pan with a rubber spatula. Break up the center with the spatula and turn off the heat. About every 30 seconds, gently pushed the cooked egg to the center of the pan and gently break up and fold the mixture.

4. Asparagus: While the eggs are cooking, place the asparagus into the microwave and cook on high power for about 2 minutes.

5. Serve: Place one cube steak on each plate, add half the asparagus and season with salt and pepper. Place half the cheesy eggs on top and season with salt and pepper.

Lunch

Keto Pork Chops

(272 calories per serving, 9.5g fat, 6g net carbs, 34g protein)

Serves 2

Ingredients

- 1 medium star anise
- 4 halved garlic cloves
- 1 T almond flour
- 1½ tsp Sambal Chili Paste
- 1 tsp sesame Oil
- ½ tsp black peppercorns
- 4 boneless pork chops
- 1 stalk lemongrass (peeled and diced)
- 1 T Fish Sauce
- 1½ tsp sugar free ketchup
- 1½ tsp soy sauce
- ½ tsp Five Spice

Directions

1. Pound the pork chops to ½-inch thick chunks on a flat work surface, using a rolling pin wrapped in wax paper.

2. Slice your garlic cloves into two, and set them aside. Purse the star anise and peppercorns in a blender and blend to a fine powder. Add the garlic and lemongrass, and then blend or pound until it forms a puree. Mix in the fish sauce, sesame oil, soy sauce, and five-spice powder.

3. Transfer the pork chops to a tray, and then add the marinade. Turn to coat, then cover and marinate for 1 to 2 hours at room temperature.

4. Preheat a pan, and coat your pork chops lightly with almond flour. Toss the chops into the pan, and allow to sear on both sides, about 2 minutes for each side or until they form a golden crust. Remove from heat and place on a cutting board.

5. Slice the chops into several strips. For the sauce, stir together the sugar free ketchup and sambal chili paste.

6. Serve with crisp garlic parmesan green beans.

Avocado Tuna Melt Bites

(135 calories, 11.8g fat, 0.8g carbs, 6.2g protein)

Serves 12

Ingredients

- 10 oz. Canned Tuna, drained
- ¼ cup Mayonnaise
- 1 medium Avocado, cubed
- ¼ cup Parmesan Cheese
- 1/3 cup Almond Flour
- ½ tsp. Garlic Powder
- ¼ tsp. Onion Powder
- Salt and Pepper to Taste
- ½ cup Coconut Oil for frying (1/4 cup absorbed)

Directions

1. Drain a can of tuna and add it to a large container where you'll be able to mix everything together.

2. Add mayonnaise, parmesan cheese, and spices to the tuna and mix together well.

3. Slice an avocado in half, remove the pit, and cube the inside. Add avocado to the tuna mixture and fold together, trying not to mash the avocado into the mixture.

4. Form the tuna mixture into balls and add roll into almond flour, cover completely. Set aside.

5. Heat coconut oil in a pan over medium heat. Once hot, add tuna balls and fry until crisp on all sides. Remove from pan and serve.

Broccoli Chicken Zucchini

(476.5 calories per serving, 34g fats, 5g carbs, 30g protein)

Serves 2

Ingredients

- 10 oz. zucchini (2 large zucchini, hallowed out)
- 2 T butter
- 3 oz. shredded cheddar cheese
- 1 cup broccoli
- 6 oz. shredded rotisserie chicken
- 2 T sour cream
- 1 stalk green onion
- Salt and pepper to taste

Directions

1. Preheat the oven to 400F and cut the zucchini in half lengthwise. The longer the zucchini the better for this recipe.

2. Using a spoon, scoop out most of the zucchini until you're left with a shell about ½-1 cm thick.

3. Pour 1 tablespoon melted butter into each zucchini boat, season with salt and pepper and place them in the oven. This allows the zucchini to cook down a little while you prepare the filling. This should take about 20 minutes.

4. Shred your rotisserie chicken using two forks to pull the meat apart. Measure out 6 oz. and put the rest in the refrigerator for another meal. A chicken, bacon, and ranch salad is perfect for lunch!

5. Cut up your broccoli florets until they're bite sized.

6. Combine the chicken and broccoli with sour cream to keep them moist and creamy. Season in this step as well.

7. Once the zucchini has had a chance to cook, take them out and add your chicken and broccoli filling.

8. Sprinkle cheddar cheese over the top of your chicken and broccoli and pop them back into the oven for an additional 10-15 minutes or until the cheese is melted and browning.

9. Garnish with chopped green onion and enjoy with more sour cream or mayonnaise.

Snacks

Cheesy Bacon Bombs

(89 calories per bacon bomb, 7.2 g fat, 0.6 net carbs, 5 g protein)

Serves 20

Ingredients

- ¼ cup almond flour
- 3 T psyllium husk powder
- ¼ tsp salt
- 1/8 tsp garlic powder
- 10 bacon slices
- 8 oz. mozzarella cheese
- ¼ cup butter, melted
- 1 large egg
- ¼ tsp freshly ground black pepper
- 1/8 teaspoon onion powder
- 1 cup of oil, lard or tallow (for frying)

Directions

1. Place 4 oz. of mozzarella cheese in a bowl. Slide ¼ cup of butter in a microwave for 15 to 20 seconds or until it melts completely.

2. Microwave the cheese until melted and gooey, about 45 to 60 seconds. Beat the butter and one egg, and then mix well. Add 3 tablespoons of psyllium husk and ¼ cup of almond flour, and the remaining spices to the mixture. Mix everything together and transfer onto a silpat.

3. Roll out the dough, or form it into a rectangle using your hands. Spread the remaining cheese over ½ of the dough, and then fold it over lengthwise. Fold again vertically to form a square shape. Using your fingers, crimp the edges, and then press the dough into a rectangle. The filling should seal tightly.

4. Slice the dough into twenty squares using a knife. Slice each bacon into two, and then place the square at the end of each piece of bacon. Roll out the dough tightly into the bacon until the ends overlap. If you need to, you can stretch the bacon before rolling. Secure the bacon with a toothpick after rolling it. Repeat for all the pieces of dough you need to end up with twenty cheesy bacon bombs.

5. Heat up the tallow, lard or oil to 350 to 375 degrees F, and then toss in the bacon bombs three to four pieces at a time to fry. Remove from heat and place on a paper towel to drain. Allow to cool completely, and then serve.

Pesto Keto Crackers

Serves 6

(210 calories per serving, 20g fat, 3g net carbs, 5g protein)

Ingredients

- 1 ¼ cup almond flour
- ¼ tsp. black pepper
- ½ tsp. salt
- ½ tsp. baking powder
- ¼ tsp. basil
- Pinch of cayenne
- 1 clove garlic
- 2 T pesto
- 3 T butter

Directions

1. Preheat oven to 325F. Line a cookie sheet with parchment paper.

2. In a medium bowl, combine almond flour, pepper, salt and baking powder and whisk until smooth.

3. Add basil, cayenne, and garlic and stir until evenly combined.

4. Next, add in the pesto and whisk until the dough forms into coarse crumbs.

5. Cut the butter into the cracker mixture with a fork or your fingers until the dough forms into a ball.

6. Transfer the dough onto the prepared cookie sheet and spread out the dough thinly until it's about 1 ½ mm thick. Make sure the thickness is the same throughout so that the crackers bake evenly.

7. Place the pan in the preheated oven and back for 14-17 minutes until light golden brown in color.

8. Once the dough has finished baking, remove it from the oven.

9. Cut crackers into the desired size.

Savory Pizza Fat Bombs

(210 calories per serving, 20g fat, 3g net carbs, 5g protein)

Serves 6

Ingredients

- 4 oz. Cream Cheese
- 14 slices Pepperoni
- 8 pitted Black Olives
- 2 T Sun Dried Tomato Pesto
- 2 T Fresh Basil, chopped
- Salt and Pepper to taste

Directions

1. Dice pepperoni and olives into small pieces.

2. Mix together basil, tomato pesto, and cream cheese.

3. Add the olives and pepperoni into the cream cheese and mix again.

4. Form into balls, then garnish with pepperoni, basil, and olive.

Dinner

Caveman Chili

(492 calories per serving, 35 g fat, 17 g carbs, 4 g fiber, 13 net carbs, 31 g protein)

Serves 8

Ingredients

- 2 lbs. ground pork
- 10 oz. green pepper
- 1 can diced tomatoes, drained
- Salt and pepper to taste
- 8 thickly cut bacon
- 1 medium yellow onion
- 6 oz. tomato paste
- 1 pack of McCormick original chili seasoning

Directions

1. Chop the peppers and onions, then place them in a Crockpot.

2. Brown the pork, and season with salt and pepper. Drain, allow to cool, and then put in the Crockpot.

3. Slice the bacon into small pieces, then cook, drain and cool. Add into the Crockpot.

4. Drain the tomatoes, and toss into the Crockpot.

5. Stir in the tomato sauce, and add the seasoning packet to the chili. Cook on low for 6 hours.

Prosciutto, Caramelized Onion, and Parmesan Braid

(303 calories per serving, 23g fats, 5g carbs, 21g protein)

Serves 6

Ingredients

- 1 T butter
- 1 medium yellow onion
- 1 clove garlic
- 1 T balsamic vinegar
- 2 tsp. fresh basil
- 3 oz. prosciutto
- 2 cups part-skim mozzarella
- ¾ cup almond flour
- ½ tsp. sea salt
- 1 egg
- ½ cup, 1 T. parmesan cheese
- 1 dash ground black pepper

Directions

1. Preheat oven to 375F. Have two pieces of parchment about 18 inches long, a rolling pin, and a baking sheet set aside. An insulated baking sheet works best for this recipe, but other baking sheets will work as well.

2. Heat a large skillet over medium heat, add the butter. When the butter stops foaming, add the onions. Cook onions, stirring occasionally until edges are brown and onions have caramelized.

3. Add garlic to the skillet. Cook for one minute, stirring occasionally. Pour balsamic vinegar over the onions and cook until almost completely evaporated.

4. Add prosciutto to the skillet, separating the thin slices as you put them in the skillet. Cook while stirring for about one minute. Stir in basil, then remove skillet from heat. Taste and adjust seasoning with salt and pepper. Prosciutto is salty already, so the addition of salt will probably not be necessary.

5. Prepare a double boiler and bring water in the lower part of the double boiler to a simmer. In the top part of the double boiler, add the mozzarella cheese, the almond flour, and the salt. Stir to evenly distribute.

6. Place the top part of the double boiler containing the almond flour and mozzarella mixture over the bottom part with the simmering water. Heat the mixture, stirring frequently, until the cheese melts and the mixture becomes a dough-like ball. Be careful not to burn yourself with steam escaping from the bottom part of the double boiler. Use a silicone mitt to hold the bowl while stirring.

7. Transfer the mozzarella dough to a piece of parchment paper. Knead it several times to incorporate any stray almond flour into the dough and completely mix the cheese and the almond flour. Pat the dough into an oval shape. Cover the dough with a second piece of parchment and roll out into an oblong shape about 14 X 9 inches. While rolling the dough out, you may need to straighten the top parchment, then flip the dough over and straighten the bottom parchment. This prevents wrinkles in the dough.

8. Spread the filling along the middle third of the dough, being careful to leave about one third of the dough on both sides. Sprinkle ½ cup of the parmesan cheese over the filling.

9. Cut approximately 1" wide strips down the sides going to where the filling starts. Make sure there's an equal number of strips on each side. Crisscross the strips. Before you get to the end, fold the bottom over the filling and cross the last few strips over top. This gives the loaf a neat and tidy end.

10. Break the egg into a small bowl. Whisk lightly and brush over the bread. (You won't use the entire egg.) Sprinkle the loaf with reserved parmesan cheese and a pinch of freshly ground black pepper on top.

11. Using the parchment the bread is already on, slide bread onto a baking sheet. Bake in preheated oven for 18-22

minutes or until it's golden brown. Let bread cool 5 minutes on the baking sheet, then transfer it to a cutting board using the parchment. Gently remove parchment from underneath, if desired. Tearing the parchment will make this process easier. Slice and serve hot with olive oil for dipping if desired.

Skilled Browned Chicken with Creamy Greens

(446 calories per serving, 38.2g fat, 2.6g carbs, 18.4g protein)

Serves 4

Ingredients

- 1 lb. chicken thighs, boneless but skin on
- 2 T coconut oil
- 1 cup chicken stock
- 1 cup cream
- 1tsp. Italian herbs
- 2 cups dark leafy greens
- 2 T butter, melted
- 2 T coconut flour
- Salt and pepper, to taste

Directions

1. Preheat a large skillet on a medium-high setting. Add two tablespoons of coconut oil to the pan. Season both sides of the chicken thighs with salt and pepper while the oil heats up. Brown chicken thighs in the skillet.

2. Fry both sides until the chicken is cooked through and crispy. While the thighs are cooking, you should start the sauce.

3. To create the sauce, melt two tablespoons of butter in a sauce pan. Once the butter stops sizzling, whisk in two tablespoons of coconut flour to form a thick paste.

4. Whisk in one cup of cream and bring the mixture to a boil. The mixture should thicken after a few minutes. Stir in the teaspoon of Italian herbs.

5. Remove cooked chicken thighs from the skillet and set aside. Pour the cup of chicken stock into the chicken skillet and deglaze the pan. Whisk in the cream sauce. Stir the greens into the pan so that they become coated with the sauce.

6. Lay the chicken thighs back on top of the greens, then remove from the heat and serve.

Dessert

Raspberry Fudge Sauce

(114 calories per serving, 11.2 g fat, 4.2 g carbs, 1.3 g fiber, 3 g net carbs, 1 g protein)

Serves 10

Ingredients

- 3.5 oz. chocolate bar, chopped (90% chocolate)
- ¼ cup heavy cream
- 4 oz. softened cream cheese
- ¼ cup erythritol
- 2 T sugar free Raspberry Syrup

Directions

1. Put the chopped chocolate and cream cheese in a double boiler, and stir well until it melts. Stir in the sweetener until smooth and fully incorporated. Remove from heat and set aside to cool.

2. Mix in the syrup and heavy cream until thick and smooth. Refrigerate for at least one hour or until it sets then serve.

Mexican Chocolate Pudding

(180 calories per serving, 15g fat, 3.5g carbs, 3g protein)

Serves 2

Ingredients

- 1 avocado
- 2½ T raw cocoa powder
- 1/16 tsp ground cayenne pepper
- 1 tsp Ceylon cinnamon
- 1 T coconut milk
- 1 T sweetener (coconut sugar, agave, maple syrup or erythritol)
- ½ tsp pure vanilla extract
- 1 pinch Stevia
- 1 pinch pink Himalayan sea salt

Directions

1. Cut and pit an avocado and blend it in a food processor until smooth.

2. Add in cocoa powder, coconut milk and vanilla extract. Blend until smooth.

3. Add in your favorite sweetener, cinnamon, a bit of stevia and ground cayenne pepper.

4. Keep blending and scraping down the sides of the food processor to get all the chunks even combined.

5. Serve with a sprinkle of coarse Himalayan pink sea salt for a flavorful crunch.

Salted Almond and Coconut Bark

(173 calories per serving, 15.7g fat, 3.5g carbs, 2.8g protein)
Serves 12

Ingredients

- ½ cup almonds
- ½ cup unsweetened flaked coconut
- ½ cup dark chocolate
- ½ cup coconut butter
- ½ tsp almond extract (optional)
- 10 drops liquid stevia (optional)
- ¼ tsp sea salt

Directions

1. Preheat oven to 350F. Spread the almonds and coconut onto a foil-lined baking sheet. Place it in the preheated oven and toast for 5-8 minutes. Stir once or twice to prevent burning. Once everything is toasted, set the baking sheet off to the side to cool.

2. In a double boiler, melt the dark chocolate and stir in the coconut butter once it has melted some. Add in the almond extract and liquid stevia (optional). Mix well and set aside.

3. Line a baking sheet with parchment or wax paper and pour the chocolate mixture in. Spread it out evenly using the back of a spoon or silicone spatula.

4. Scatter the toasted almond and coconut flakes over the top and press gently with your hands so that everything is touching the chocolate. Sprinkle lightly with sea salt and let it set in the refrigerator for at least an hour.

5. Once it has set, slice with a knife or pizza roller.

Conclusion

I'd like to thank you for getting this book and reading it all the way to the end!

It's such a shame that we're so used to consuming high carbohydrate foods that the thought of reducing your carbohydrate intake seems impossible. While our bodies need some carbohydrates to function, the amount of carbohydrates we consume is too much, and this is what has led to many people being overweight. Reducing your carbohydrate intake to put your body in the ketosis state where it burns fat for energy is what you'll need for long-term weight loss. While adapting to the ketogenic diet is possible, remember that you're going to experience withdrawal symptoms when you begin, as I indicated earlier. However, over time, things will become much easier.

I hope this book helped you learn more about the ketogenic diet and make the necessary dietary changes for a better you.

Should you find this book extremely of help, sharing it with your friends and loved ones will be greatly valued.

Go to http://bit.ly/ketoreview to review and thanks in advance for any kind of support!

Thank you and good luck!

- *Sandra*

Would You Like to Know More?

To check what are The 101 Tips That Burn Belly Fat Daily go to my page here:

=> http://projecteasylife.com/101tips <=

To see what are The 7 (Quick & Easy) Cooking Tricks To Banish Your Boring Diet go to my website here:

=> http://projecteasylife.com/7-tricks <=

[BONUS]

Preview of My Other Book, Wheat Belly Diet

(…)

Why Use the Wheat Belly Diet for the Best Results?

If you have tried and failed with other diets, perhaps you were not eliminating the right types of foods. Rethinking wheat has helped people to eliminate the harm it causes to your body. Getting rid of belly fat has thus far been a successful goal for people using the Wheat-Belly Diet.

Very few wheat-based foods are actually healthy for you to eat. The wheat used today, which Dr. Davis calls "Frankenwheat", is genetically modified, and it isn't the same wheat that your parents used to eat.

The modification of the wheat plant has allowed it to be thicker and shorter, so that it is more beneficial for farmers, and more resistant to disease. The bad aspect of this wheat is that it is not as nutritionally rich as conventional wheat, and can damage your health.

The glycemic index is higher in today's wheat than it is in sugar. Some candy bars have a healthier glycemic index than a slice of wheat bread. Glutens that are present in larger amounts in today's wheat cause cravings, and that leads to excess belly fat.

Dr. Davis says that you can expect better results from a wheat-free meal plan, because wheat is more than simply a gluten source. "Frankenwheat" affects the mind, by stimulating your appetite and it can cause depression and anxiety, especially for people who are overweight.

Giving up wheat will allow you to lose belly fat, and can also help in other health issues, such as those mentioned above. People are finally beginning to see the negative effects of today's wheat on their health, and those who stay with the Wheat Belly Diet often find benefits that they did not even expect.

(…)

To check out the rest of the book *Wheat Belly Diet*, go to Amazon here: http://bit.ly/wheatbellydiet

Check Out My Other Books

Below you'll find some of my other books that are popular on Amazon and Kindle as well. Simply go to the links below to check them out. Alternatively, you can visit my author page on Amazon to see other work done by me:

Author page: http://bit.ly/SandraWilliams

Gluten Free And Wheat Free Total Health Revolution

Wheat Belly Cookbook – *37 Wheat Free Recipes To Lose The Wheat And Have All-Day Energy* (http://bit.ly/bellycookbook)

Gluten Free – *The Gluten Free Diet For Beginners Guide, What Is Celiac Disease, How To Eat Healthier And Have More Energy* (http://bit.ly/glutenfreebook)

Gluten Free Cookbook – *30 Healthy And Easy Gluten Free Recipes For Beginners, Gluten Free Diet Plan For A Healthy Lifestyle* (http://bit.ly/gfreecookbook)

How To REALLY Set And Achieve Goals

Goals – *Setting And Achieving S.M.A.R.T. Goals, How To Stay Motivated And Get Everything You Want From Your Life Faster* (http://bit.ly/getsmartgoals)

Prevent And Reverse Diabetes Disease

Diabetic Cookbook – *30 Diabetes Diet Recipes For Diabetic Living, Control Low Sugar And Reverse Diabetes Naturally* (http://bit.ly/diabetic-cookbook)

Get Healthy, Have More Energy And Live Longer With Natural Paleo And Mediterranean Foods

Paleo – *The Paleo Diet For Beginners Guide, Easy And Practical Solution For Weight Loss And Healthy Eating* (http://bit.ly/healthypaleo)

Paleo Cookbook – *30 Healthy And Easy Paleo Diet Recipes For Beginners, Start Eating Healthy And Get More Energy With Practical Paleo Approach* (http://bit.ly/tastypaleo)

Mediterranean Diet – *Easy Guide To Healthy Life With Mediterranean Cuisine, Fast And Natural Weight Loss For Beginners* (http://bit.ly/mediterraneanbook)

Mediterranean Diet Cookbook – *30 Healthy And Easy Mediterranean Diet Recipes For Beginners* (http://bit.ly/mediterracookbook)

Extremely Fast Weight Loss With Low Carb Approach

Ketogenic Diet Cookbook – *30 Keto Diet Recipes For Beginners, Easy Low Carb Plan For A Healthy Lifestyle And Quick Weight Loss* (http://bit.ly/ketocookbook)

Atkins Cookbook – *30 Quick And Easy Atkins Diet Recipes For Beginners, Plan Your Low Carb Days With The New Atkins Diet Book* (http://bit.ly/atkinscookbook)

Amazing Weight Loss Tips, Tricks And Motivation

Weight Loss – *30 Tips On How To Lose Weight Fast Without Pills Or Surgery, Weight Loss Motivation And Fat Burning Strategies* (http://bit.ly/weightlosstipsbook)

Ultimate Guide To Diets – *Choose The Best Diet For Your Body, Live Healthy And Happy Life Without Supplements And Pills* (http://bit.ly/dietsbook)

The Obesity Cure – *How To Lose Weight Fast And Overcome Obesity Forever* (http://bit.ly/obesitybook)

Unique Beauty Tips Every Woman Should Know

Younger Next Month – *Anti-Aging Guide For Women* (http://bit.ly/beyoungerbook)

Hair Care And Hair Growth Solutions – *How To Regrow Your Hair Faster, Hair Loss Treatment And Hair Growth Remedies* (http://bit.ly/haircarebook)

Improve State Of Mind, Defeat Bad Feelings And Be Happy!

Anxiety Workbook – *Free Cure For Anxiety Disorder And Depression Symptoms, Panic Attacks And Social Anxiety Relief Without Medication And Pills* (http://bit.ly/anxietybook)

The Depression Cure – *Depression Self Help Workbook, Cure And Free Yourself From Depression Naturally And For Life* (http://bit.ly/depressioncurebook)

If the links do not work, for whatever reason, you can simply search for the titles on the Amazon website to find them. Best regards!

CPSIA information can be obtained
at www.ICGtesting.com
Printed in the USA
LVOW10s2218290118
564504LV00029B/953/P